London's Low Carb Lite

Written By
Adrienne Reade

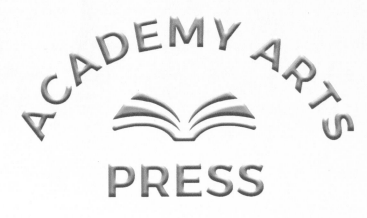

ACADEMY ARTS
PRESS

www.academyartspress.com

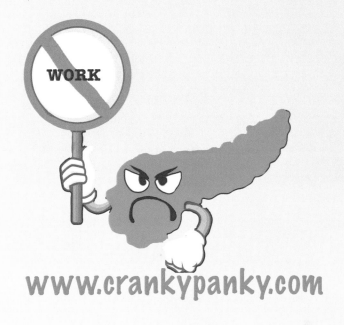

www.crankypanky.com

Illustrations By
Brandy Roy & Mandy Morreale

Hi! My name is London and I am 6 years-old.
At first glance I may look just like every other
little girl out there.
But if you look a little closer, you may notice a few things...
I wear an insulin pump and blood glucose meter.
Can you spot my devices?
It's kind of like a fun game of peek-a-boo because they move
around to different spots, like my arms and legs.

1

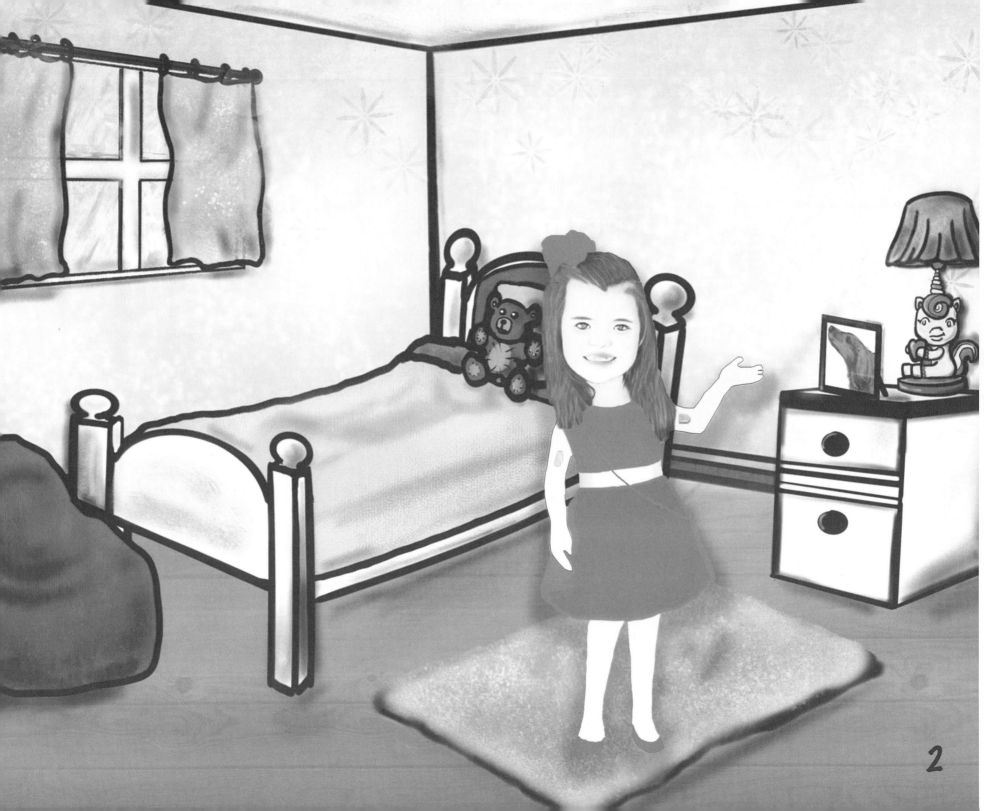

I wear these two devices to give me medicine called insulin and to monitor my blood sugar.
My Dad says I'm high tech!
I also wear a little purse that holds my diabetes supplies. I always carry my phone that controls my insulin pump, and jelly beans in case my blood sugar gets too low.
My 2 year-old brother knows about the candy too.
He loves to get a little treat from my purse.

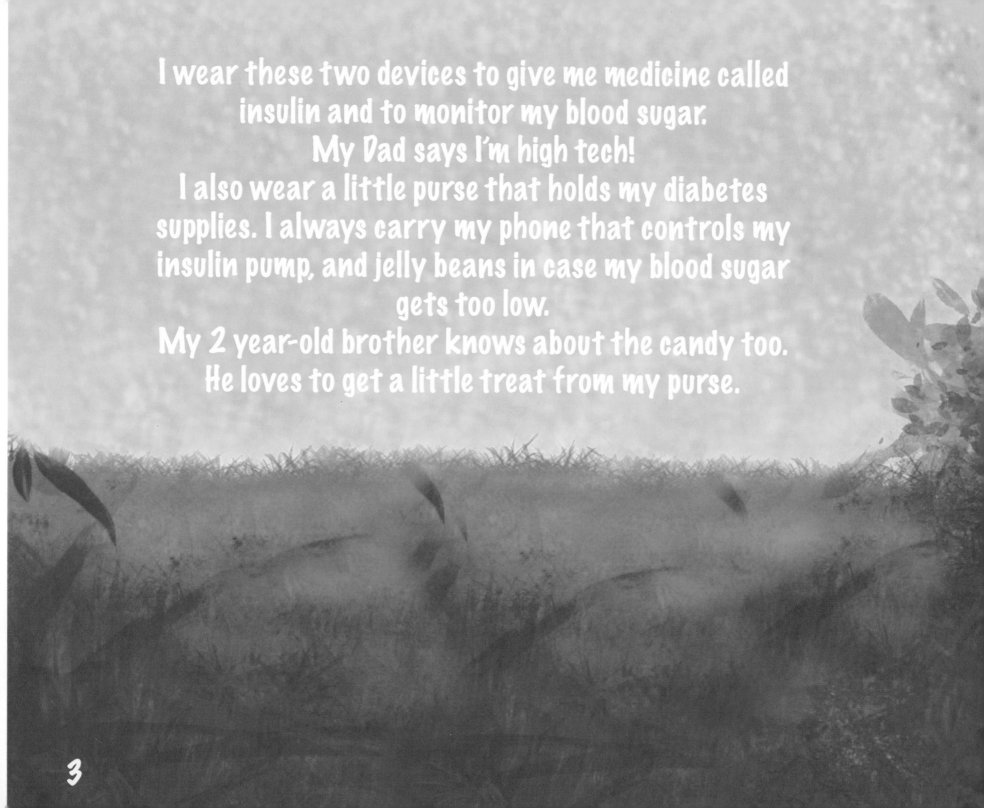

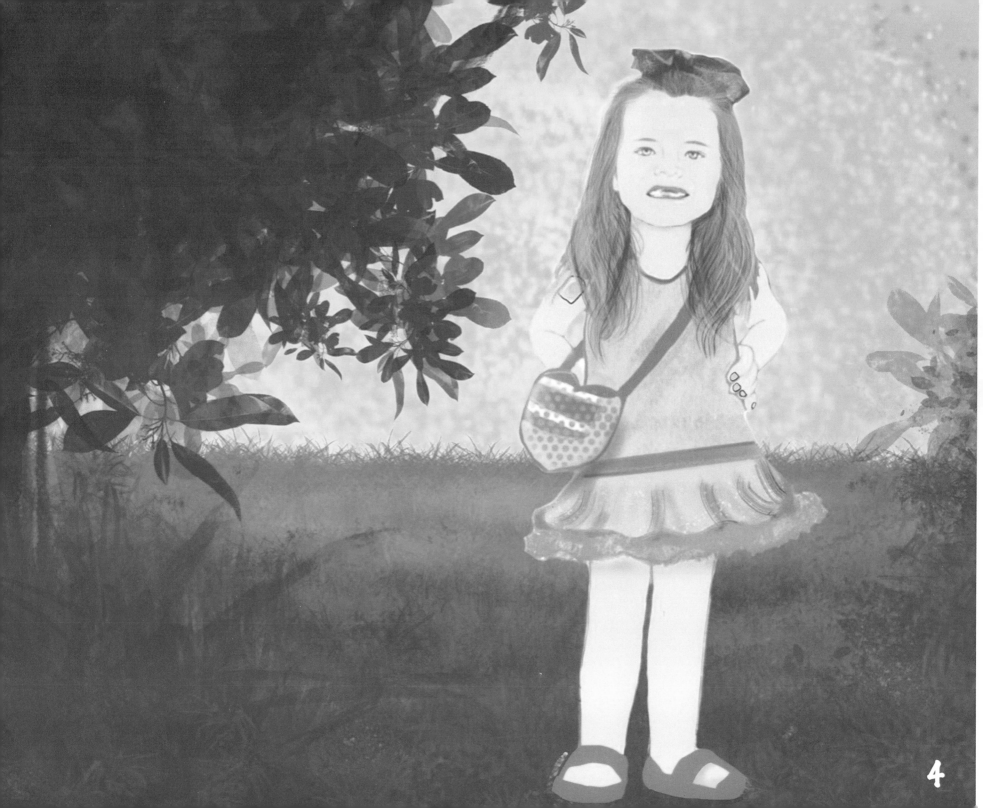

4

When I was 16-months old my Mom had a feeling that something was wrong. Luckily she noticed I was losing weight, drinking a ton of water, and I was very tired. I was very sick and had to stay in the hospital for several days. That's when I found out I had Type 1 Diabetes. I have to take shots of insulin because my body doesn't make it like it should. This means every time I eat, I need insulin, which I get through my pump.

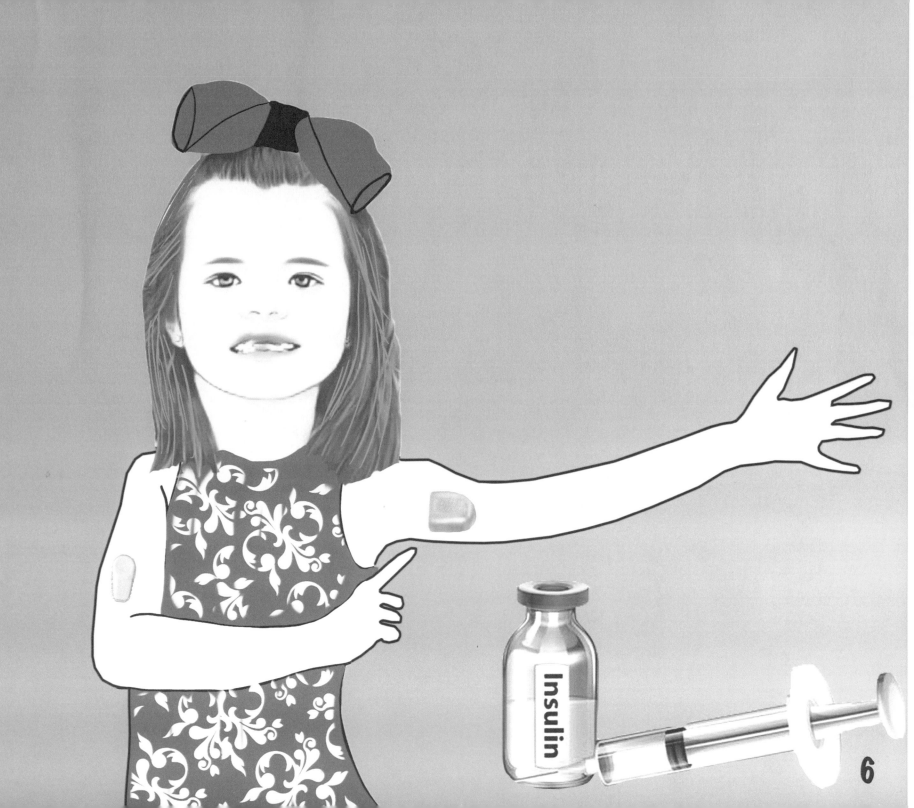

Insulin

6

When I was first diagnosed with T1D, I ate foods with lots of carbohydrates in them, like bread, sugary fruits, and potatoes. My Mom and Dad did what they were told to do by the Doctor, but my blood sugar was crazy!
Have you ever been on a roller coaster? That's what it felt like... I was high, then low, then high, then low.

I felt really sick when I was on that ride.

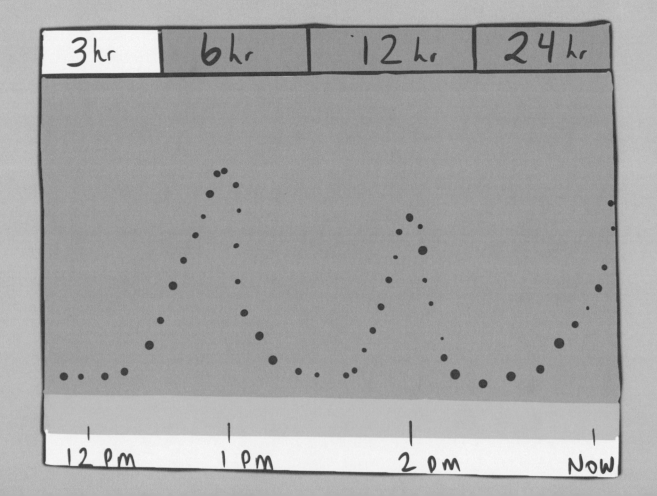

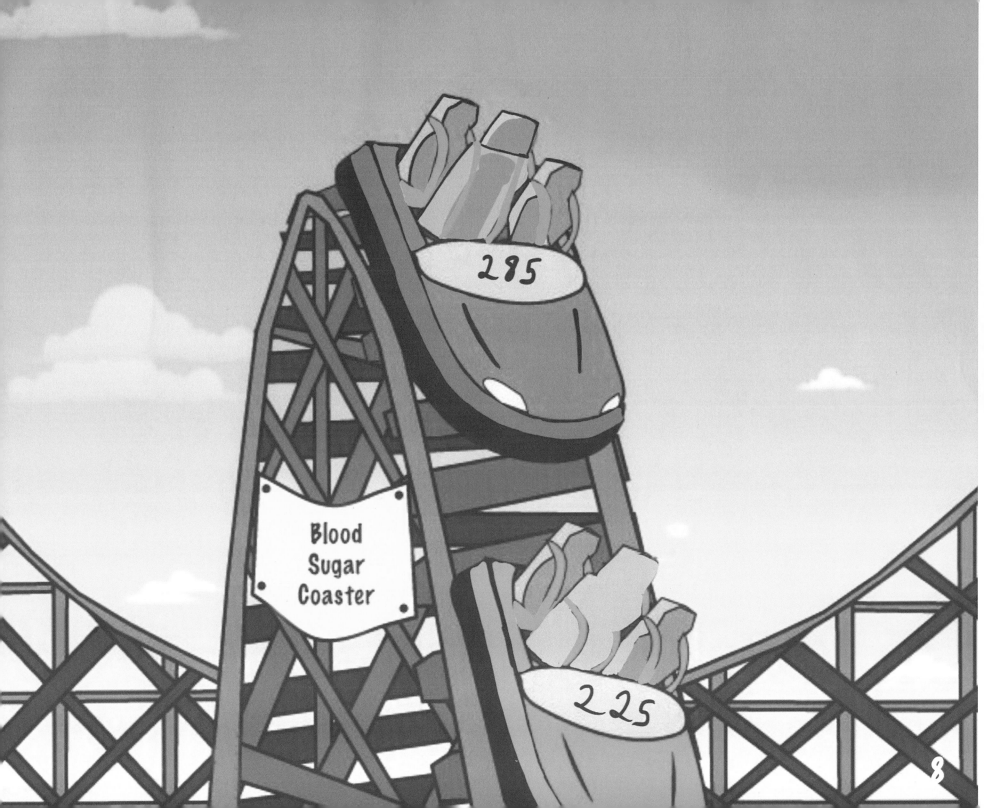

One day, my Mom said
"Hey, what if we eat less carbohydrates and use less insulin? I wonder what would happen?"
Ah ha! Maybe I could get off this roller coaster ride by eating different foods?
So I started eating the same foods that you might eat, but my Mom made sure they were safe for me.
She is great at finding alternatives that I can eat, and that make me feel amazing!
I stepped off that crazy ride for good!

DIABETES LOG BOOK

DATE: March 17 2021

TIME	BLOOD GLUCOSE	INSULIN
7:30 am	116	0.20
12:15 pm	100	0.10
5:32 pm	120	0.25

NOTES: Breakfast = low carb pancakes
Lunch: cucumber, LC pizza

Less Carbs = Less medicine!

ow carb ternatives

So you may be asking yourself,
What can I eat?
Well, I eat the same things that you do!
Pizza, chicken nuggets, fries,
and ice cream!
I can eat it all...but shhh...,don't tell anyone,
but they are low-carb versions!
Pretty much any food can be made into a
low-carb version. I can be a normal kid and
eat anything I want, but it is just made with
a few different ingredients.

Some of my favorite low-carb foods are cucumbers, cheese, and bacon! Who doesn't like bacon?! Actually, my Mom is the only person I know who doesn't like bacon! More for me! Did I mention that my family eats mostly low-carb too? Yup...the food is all so yummy that we don't miss the carbs!

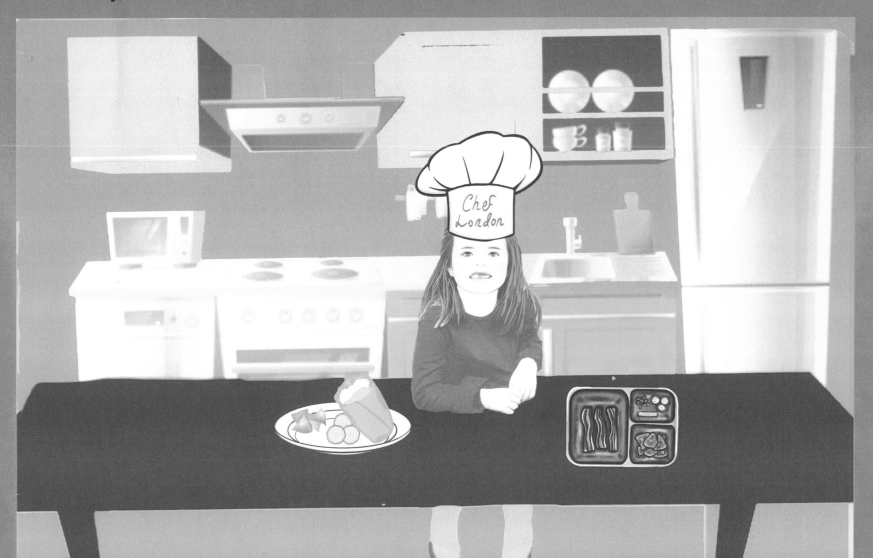

Sometimes I run around so much, or jump on the trampoline with my brothers, and my blood sugar drops too low. I have a superdog named Sherlock. He's my detective dog who can smell when I'm not quite right. High or low, he has the nose! He goes everywhere I go and wears a pack to show people that he's a working dog and not a pet. It's fun taking him places but it's hard work too! People ask to pet him, but I tell them that he's working keeping me safe. Don't worry though, he gets lots of toys, treats, and love!

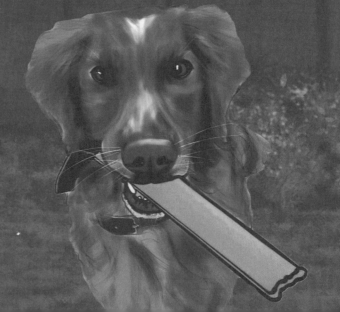

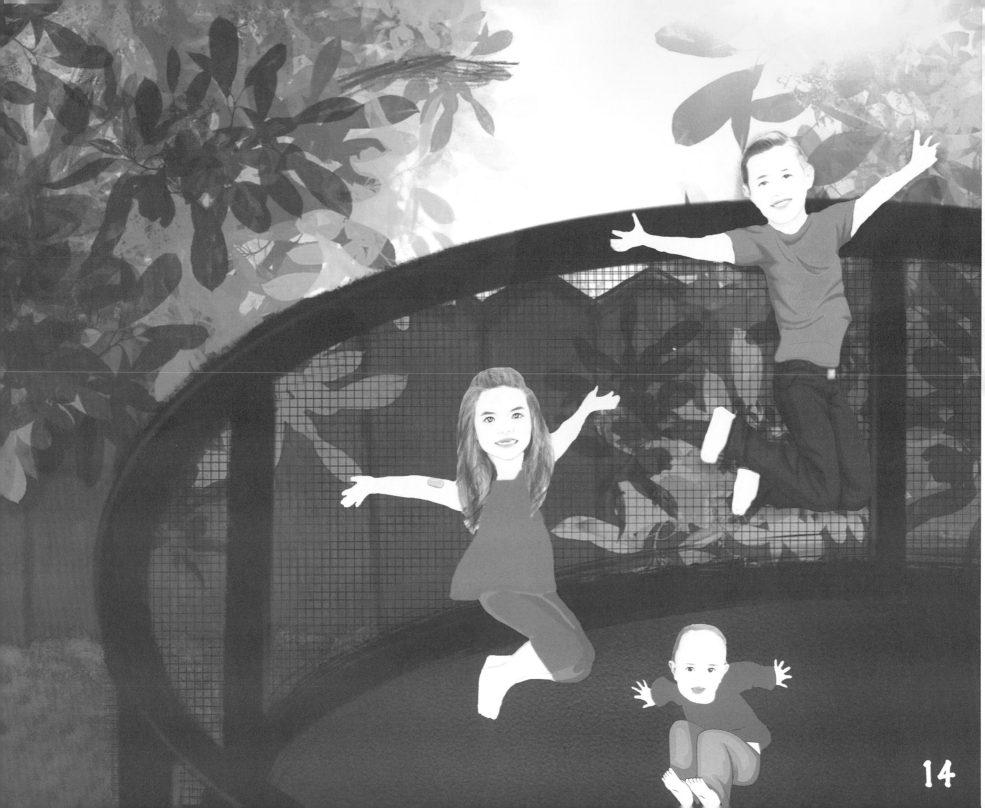

14

Every few days I have to put on a new insulin pump.
I'm really brave, but it does hurt..like a shot you get at the
doctors office. I also have to poke my fingers to check my
blood sugar. I've been doing it so long, I don't even feel it!
I can even do the test all by myself!

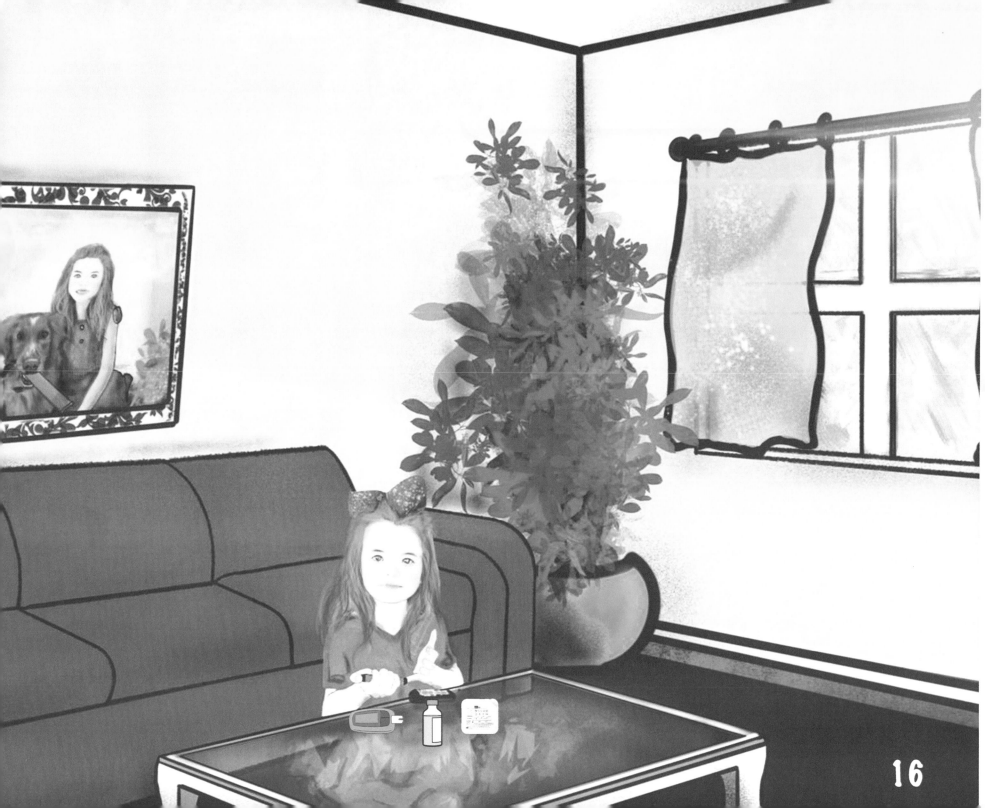

When I go to a birthday party, or an event where they serve
high-carb treats, it's not a problem for me!
I can take the bread off the sandwich, the cheese off the pizza,
and bring my own special cupcake.

I'm not at the party to eat anyway...
I just want to see my friends and play!
And those goody bag treats?
My favorite.
I just put them in my stash for when my blood sugar is low.

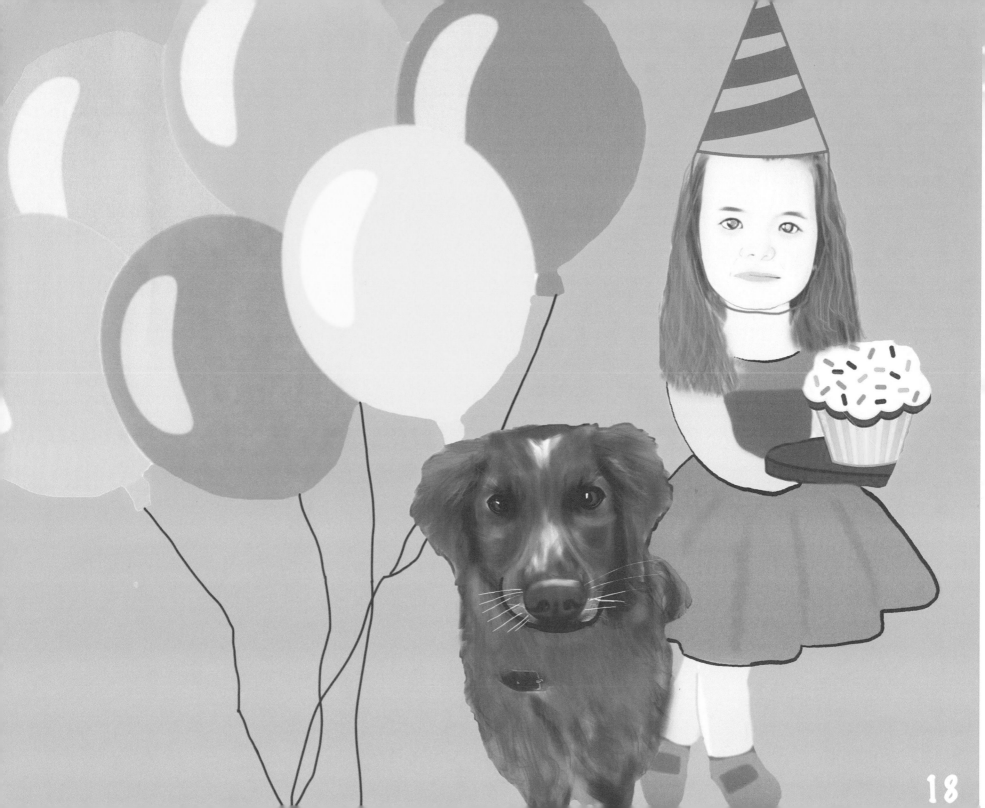

I go to school at home and my Mom is my teacher.
Since she's the one who helps me with
my diabetes it works out great!
I like to do my school at home, with my brothers.
Okay, my little brother just gets into everything,
while my Mom tries to keep him busy!

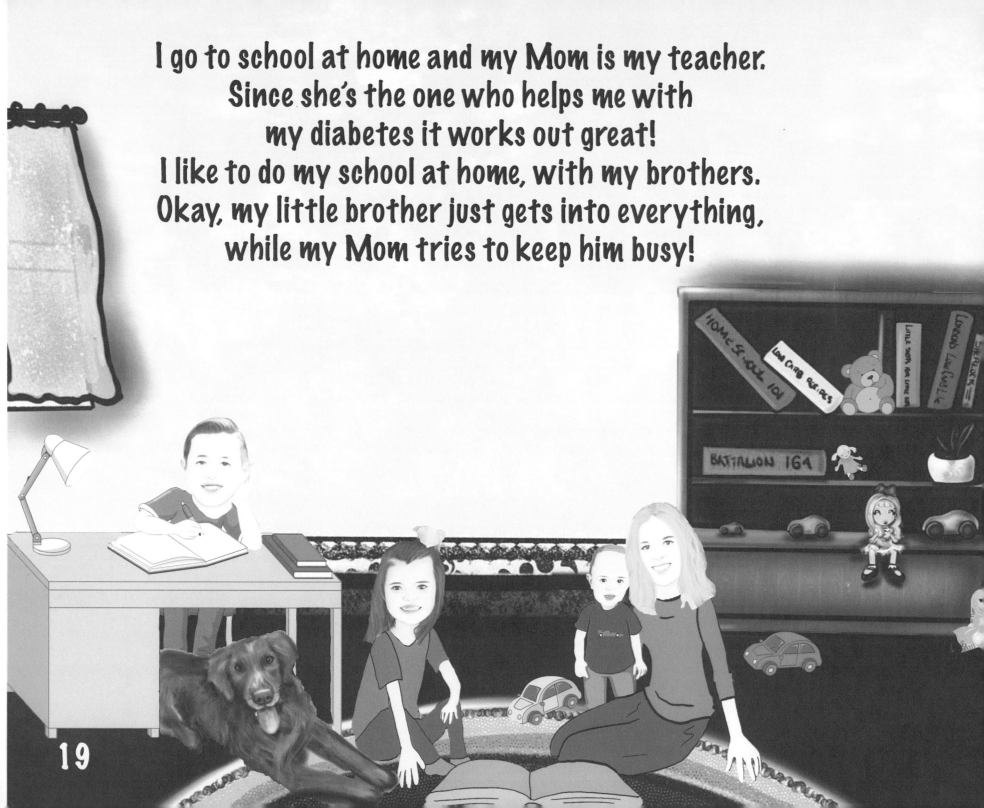

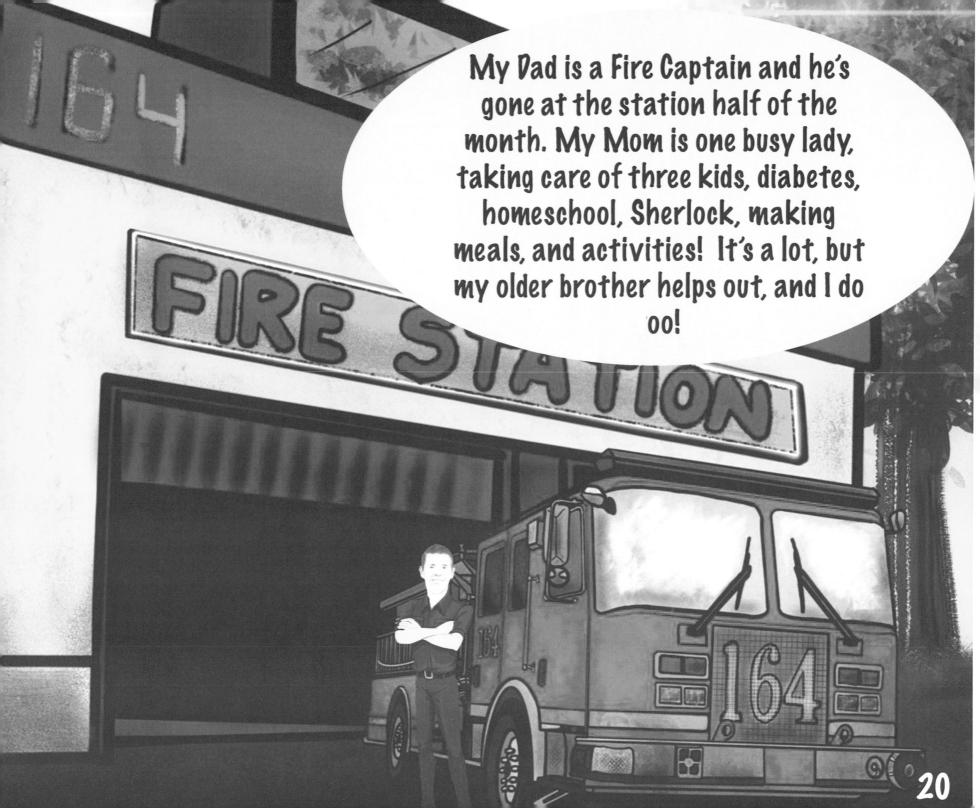

Swimming is one of my favorite things to do.
I love to jump off the rocks and go down the slide.
My Mom says I'm a daredevil!
Diabetes doesn't slow me down!
I eat lots of protein and veggies to help me grow and make me strong.

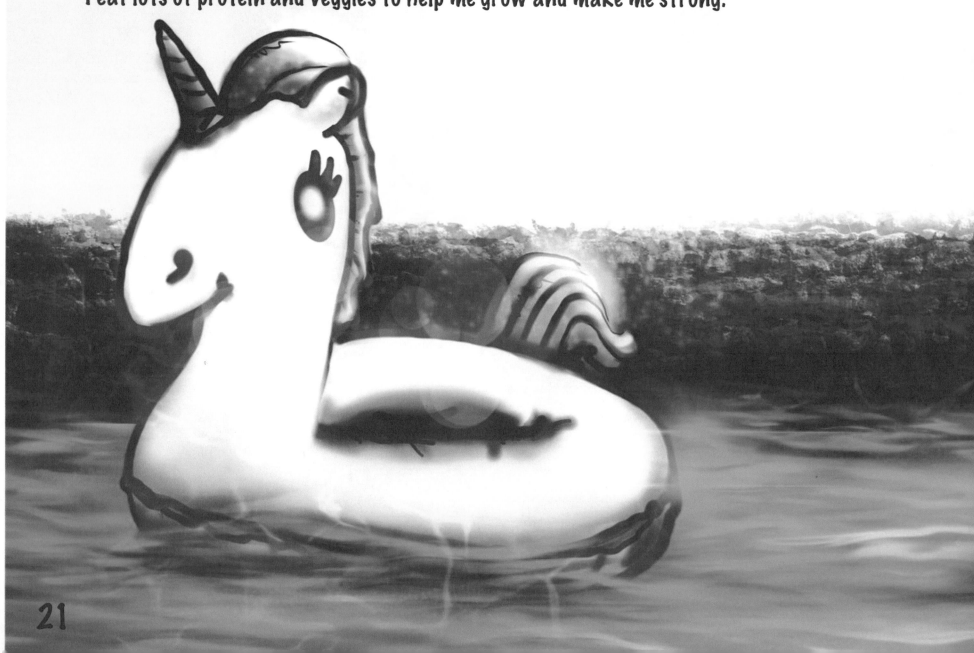

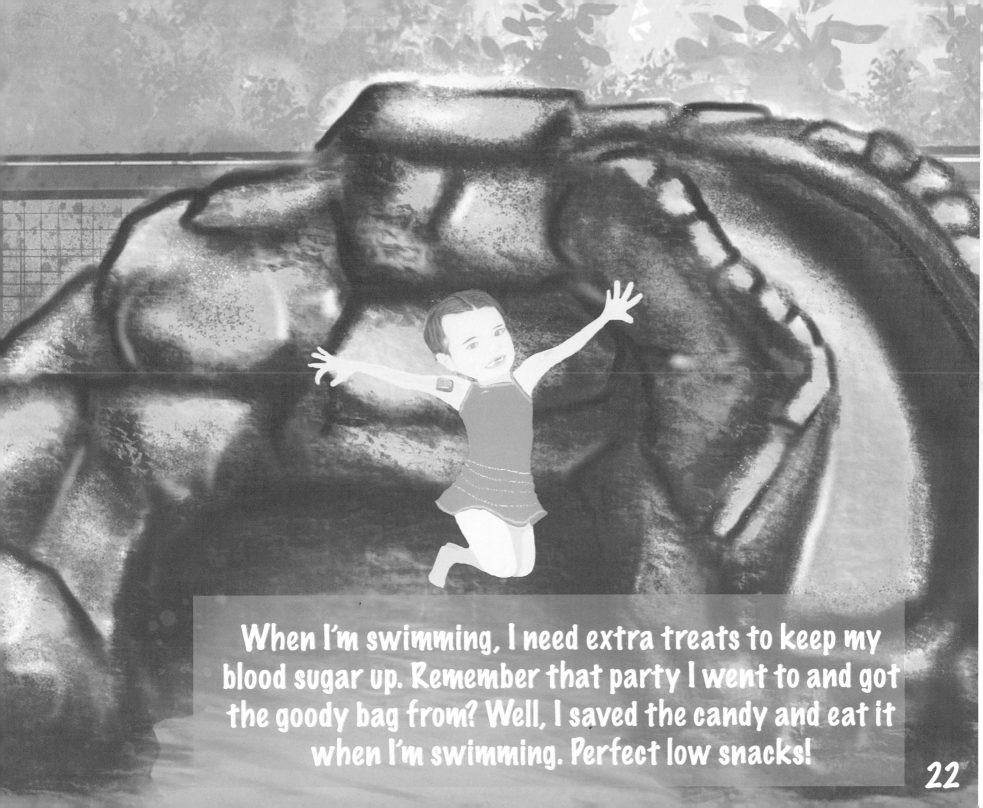

When I'm swimming, I need extra treats to keep my blood sugar up. Remember that party I went to and got the goody bag from? Well, I saved the candy and eat it when I'm swimming. Perfect low snacks!

We are a busy family and sometimes my Mom doesn't feel like cooking.
It's pretty neat that now stores sell so many low-carb, blood sugar friendly foods! Some of the foods we order can be shipped right to our front door!

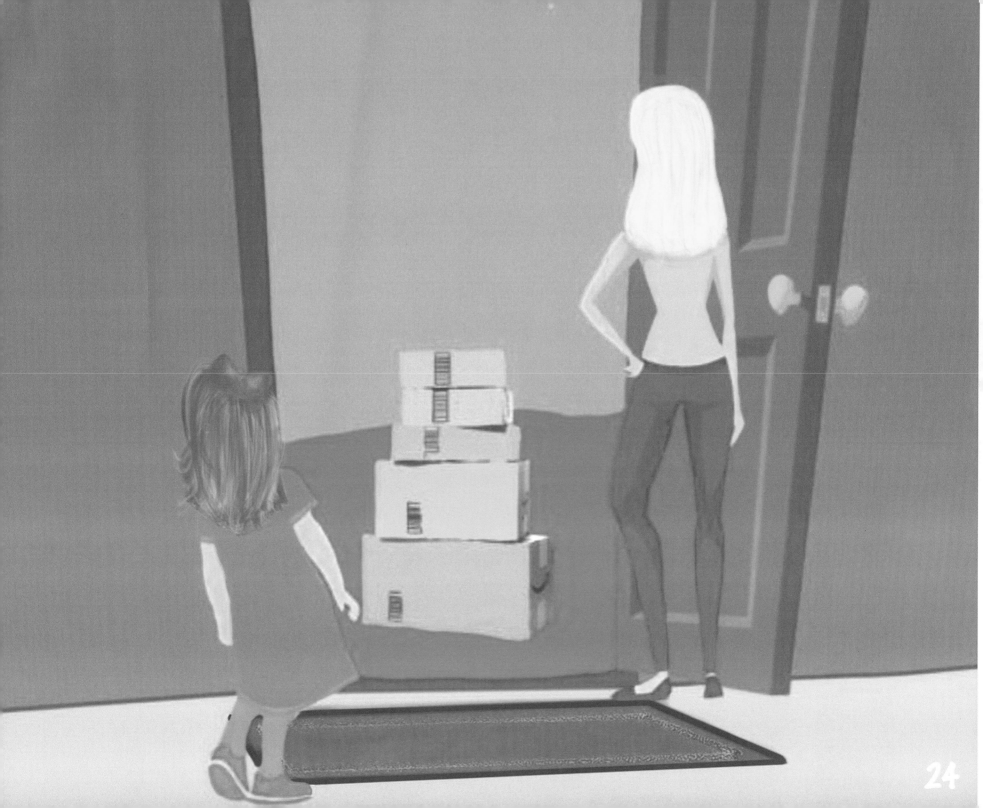

Some days diabetes doesn't play fair and my blood sugar just doesn't cooperate.
My Mom and Dad try their best, but it's a hard job being a pancreas! My pump can stop working or get ripped out, and other factors like exercise, being sick, growth, and even the weather can make my blood sugar go crazy! Days like this are hard and make me sad, but I try to have a good attitude. I have lots of friends that also have T1D, and they help me feel like I'm not alone!

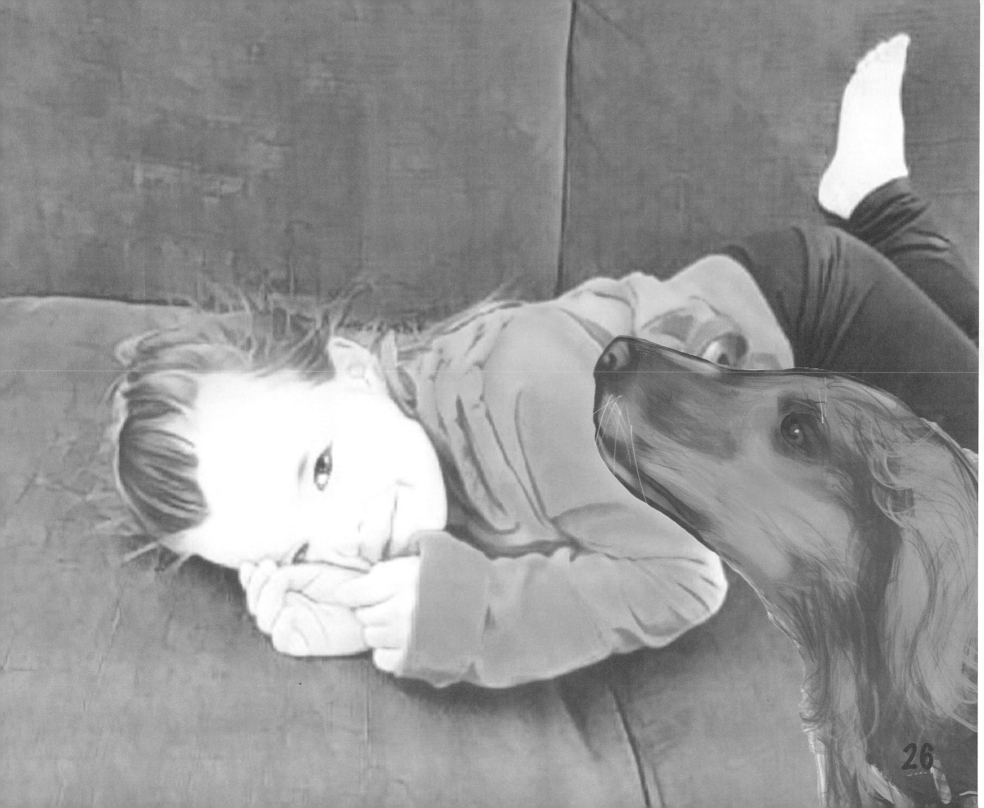

My life with T1D is just like any other kid's. I can swim and jump and play with my brothers. I get to eat pancakes, sandwiches, pizza, and ice cream, Oh and don't forget the bacon! I eat like a normal kid.

My body might be different inside, so eating my special low-carb versions work better for me. Living this way allows me to be a normal, healthy, happy kid!

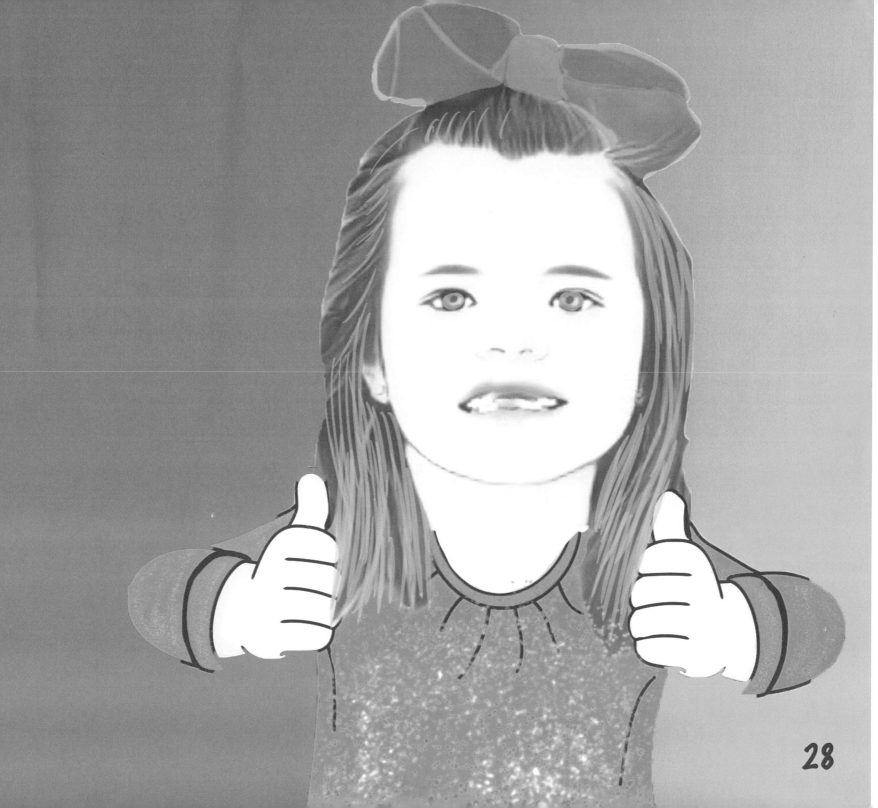

Note to caregivers/parents:

This book is not intended to provide any medical advice. Please consult your Doctor before making any changes.

Our approach is unconventional in that the standard diet for kids with T1d is high in carbs. We were told to let London eat whatever she wanted and to cover those foods with insulin. She ran much higher than we were comfortable with. Her blood sugar was all over the place, scary lows, crazy highs, she was gaining weight and we were all miserable

We did our own research, found a new Endocrinologist and decided to try low carb eating. We had almost instant success with normal blood sugar (65-120 mg/dl)! London has been low carb for almost 5 years. She is growing appropriately, is very bright and has tons of energy. Her body is fueled by protein and nutrients and her A1C has been below 5.3 since changing her diet.

For more recipes, low carb food ideas, and more about London's Low Carb Life please visit our social media pages on Facebook and Instagram. TeamLondonT1D

To London and all of the brave children and adults who fight this battle everyday.
May this invisible disease not be so invisible!

CPSIA information can be obtained
at www.ICGtesting.com
Printed in the USA
LVRC100138220421
685165LV00001B/4